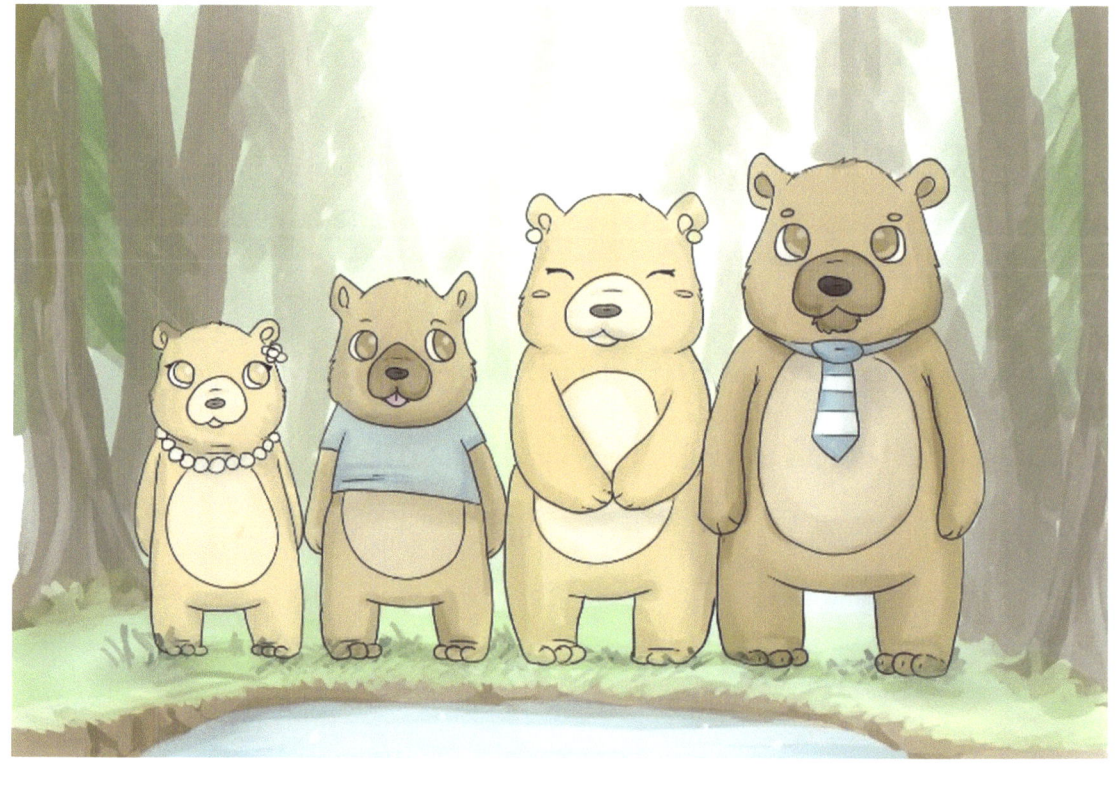

Let me tell you a story that touched my heart.

Hmm, now let's see where to start. I guess I will start with the family, theres Mama B, Daddy D then Barlow Bear and his sister Brie. They lived near some Evergreens that stretched towards the sky, close to a lake called the Tear from Gods Eye.

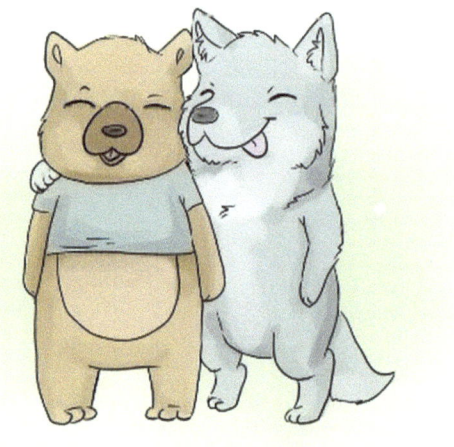

Barlows best friend was a wolf cub named Sage, those two were inseparable and around the same age. Well, one day Barlow woke up feeling sickly and weak and remained the same for days and weeks.

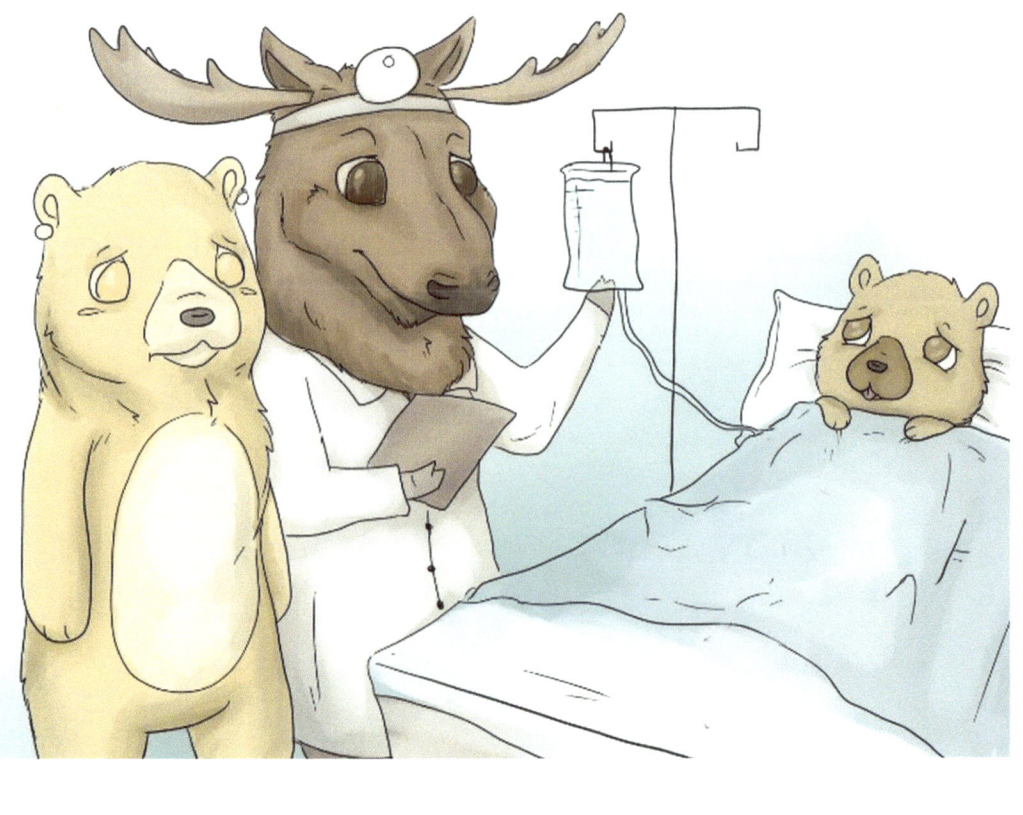

So Mama B took Barlow to the Incredible

Hospitable Animal Hospital to see a moose named Dr. Bruce so he could run test after test. She knew he was known throughout the forest for being the very best. And the work he did was not just pud work, it was high sophisticated blood work.

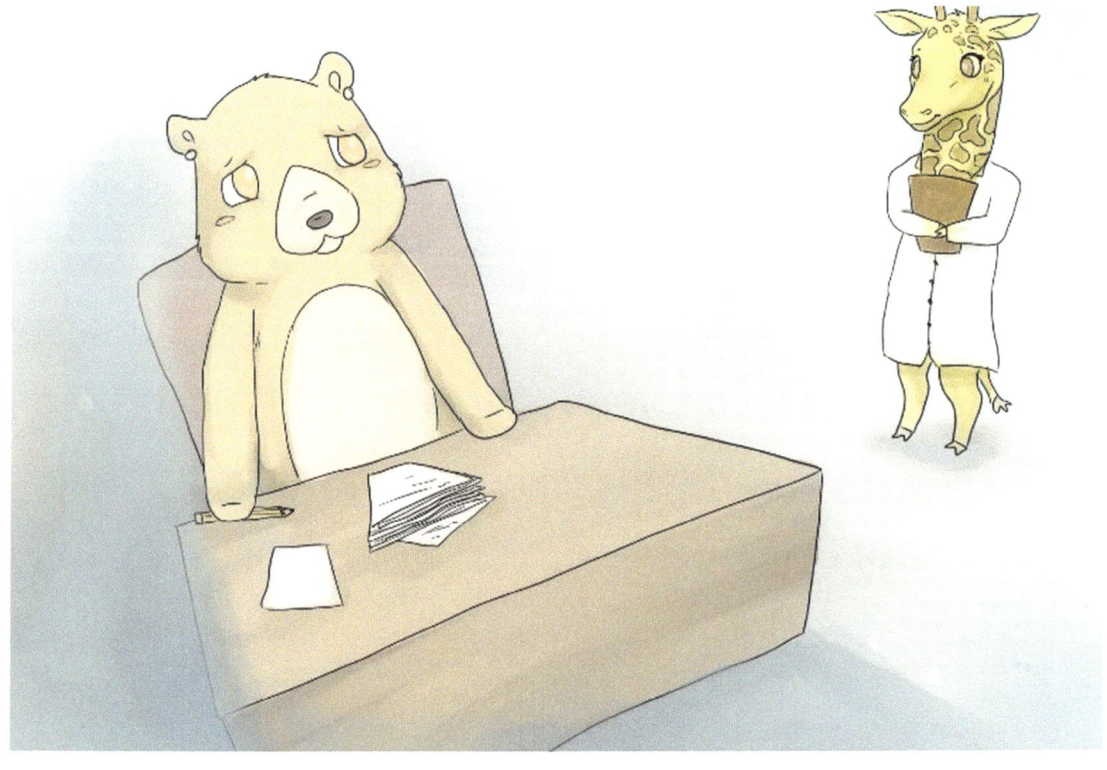

Dr. Bruce had a wonderful staff of giraffe who were as nice and gentle as a warm sponge bath. So Mama B went up to the clerk and filled out a mountain of paperwork. Then a giraffe named Dixie said at the rear end of the hospital is our proctologist, next to him in room ten, is Dr. Bruces office. Dr. Bruce was such a softy and offered them cookies, candy and coffee. While Mama B drank her cup of mud, Dr. Bruce grabbed a needle so he could draw Barlows blood.

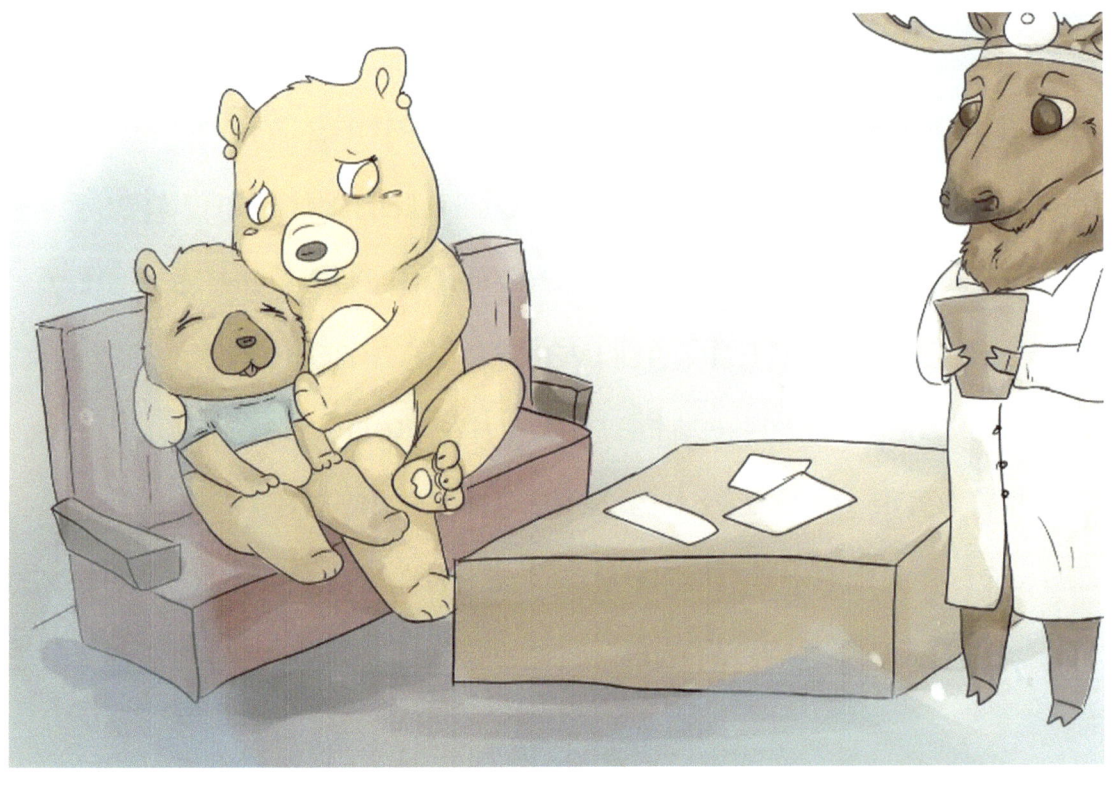

Afterwards, it was back to the waiting room where Barlow flipped through about fifteen magazines while waiting for Dr. Bruce to spill the beans. They waited and waited and waited and not knowing was something they hated. Finally he came out with a long look on his face and told them it was cancer then explained the treatment options with a soft and gentle manner.

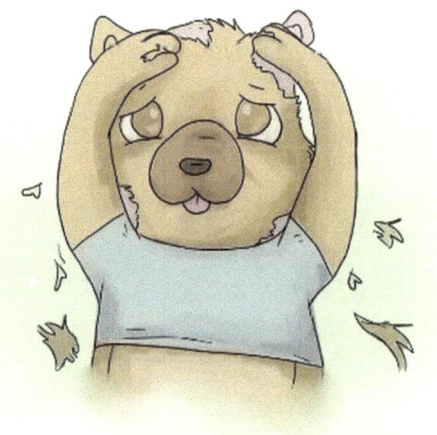

Mama B's heart fell to her knees and Barlows fertile mind turned to Swiss cheese. Although, they took the news so terribly, they collected their thoughts enough to decide on Chemotherapy. After a few months, the treatments were going well but clump after clump out his hair fell. Until one morning when getting out of bed, his last clump of hair had fallen off his head.

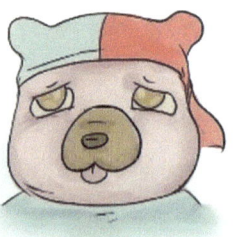
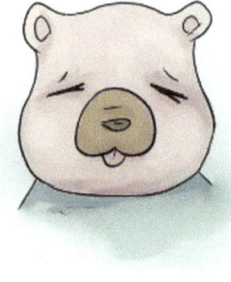
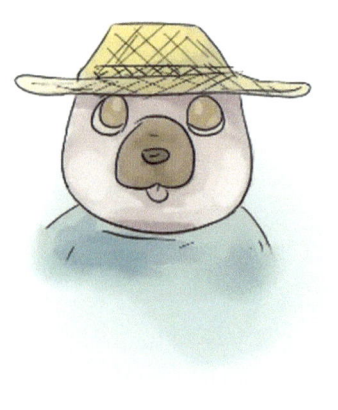

At first he tried to hide his head with a do rag, he had both a red and blue rag. Then he tried Daddy D's straw hat, but it was a much to tall hat. Finally, his problem was solved. He decided to accept the fact that the head he had was bald.

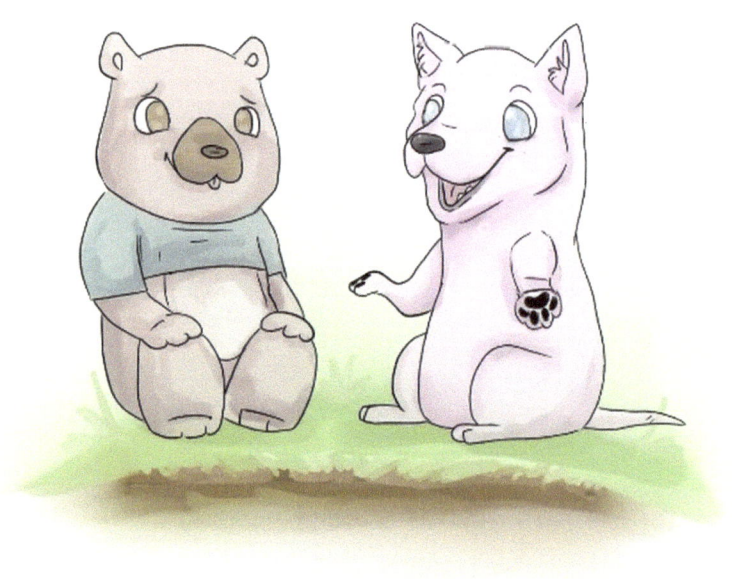

Sage accepted him just the way he was and just to show he looked okay, he got all his hair buzzed. Well, one day while Barlow and Sage were playing war they had received the news they had been praying for.

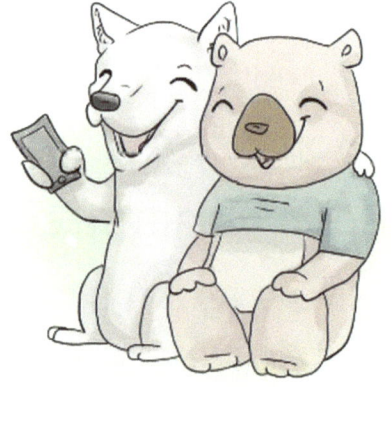

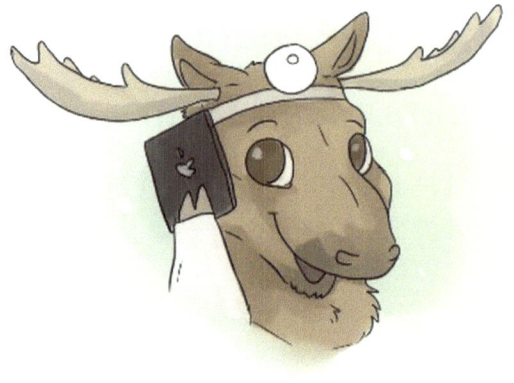

"The cancer was gone." Said Dr. Bruce on the phone. They were wrapped around happy like skin on a bone. "He is in remission." Dr. Bruce said. "He will soon regain strength and the hair on his head." So Barlow and his family went down to the lake, and bar-b-qued some ham, salmon and steak. Mama B made Barlows favorite dessert, Grubs-N-Berries A-La-Tort.

The End.

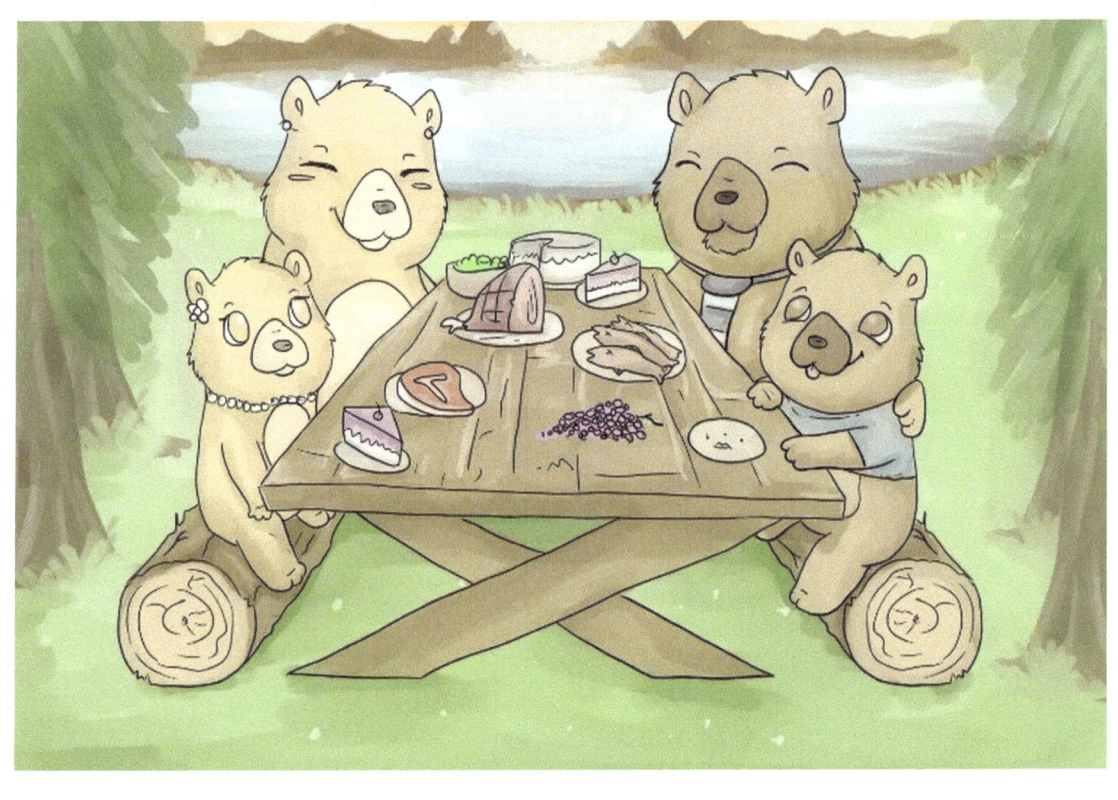